YOGA FOR SENIORS OVER 50

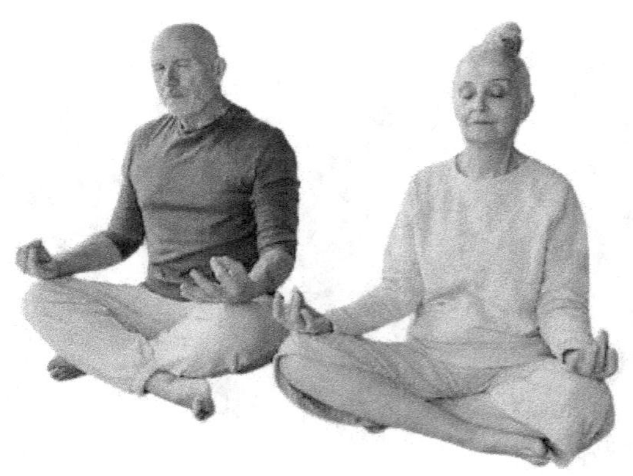

Dr. Mary Dixon

Copyright © 2023 by Dr. Mary Dixon

All rights reserved. No part of this publication may be reproduced, distributed, or transmitted in any form or by any means, including photocopying, recording, or other electronic or mechanical methods, without the prior written permission of the publisher, except in the case of brief quotations embodied in critical reviews and certain other noncommercial uses permitted by copyright law.

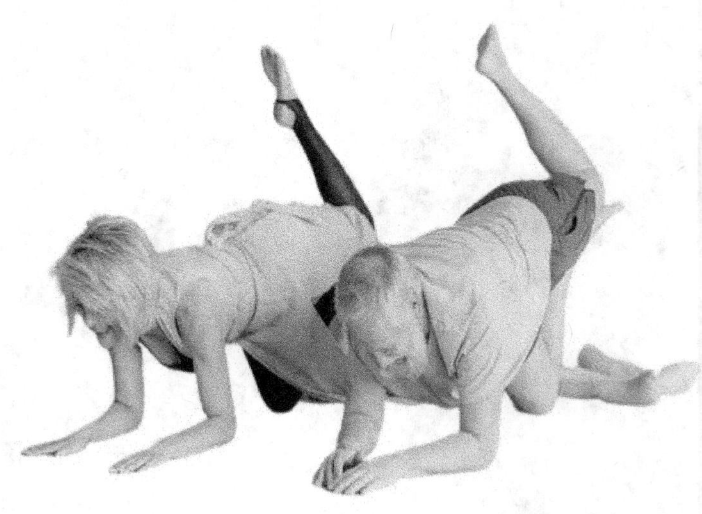

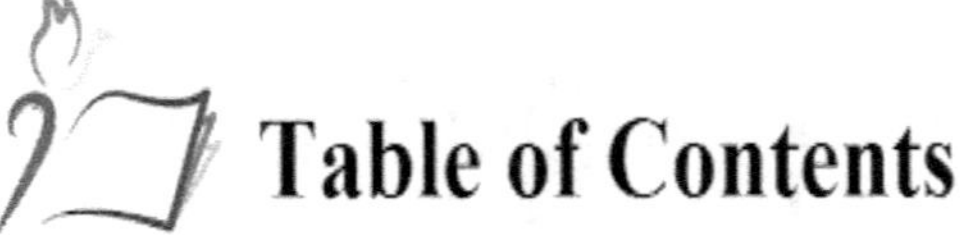

Table of Contents

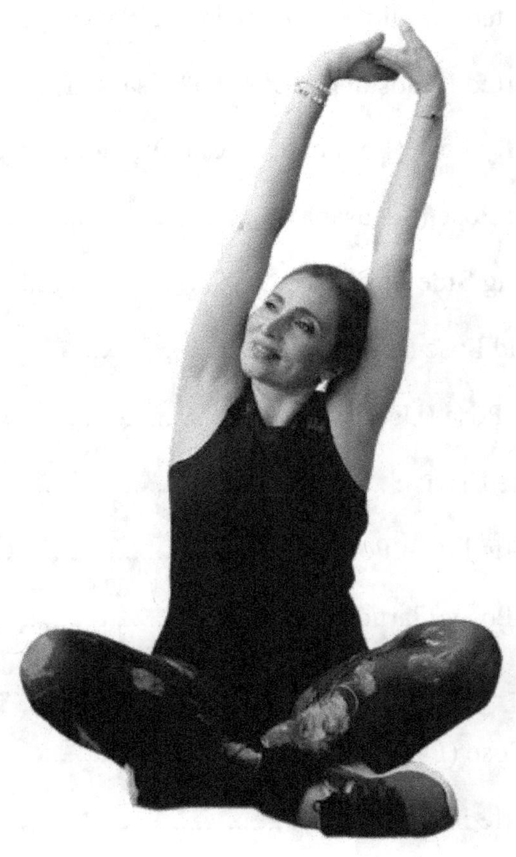

INTRODUCTION

Once upon a time in a peaceful town nestled between rolling hills, there lived a group of vibrant old souls who were forever young at heart.

They were the residents of the Golden Age Retirement Community, a place where laughter, companionship, and joy filled the air. Among the many activities that brought them together, one stood out for its remarkable impact on their lives—yoga.

Every morning, as the sun bathed the community in its warm glow, the residents gathered in the tranquil courtyard, their yoga mats unfurled and anticipation in their eyes.

Their instructor, the graceful and wise Mrs. Sharma, led them through a series of gentle stretches and soothing postures. As they moved in harmony with their breath, a profound transformation took place within each of them.

Yoga had become the secret to unlocking their bodies' dormant potential. The residents discovered newfound strength, flexibility, and balance, defying the stereotypes of old age.

With each practice, their joints loosened, muscles toned, and posture improved. They marveled at their ability to bend and twist, feeling rejuvenated with each fluid motion.

But the physical benefits were merely the surface of their yoga journey. The real magic happened within their hearts and minds.

Yoga brought them inner peace, harmony, and a deep connection to themselves. Mrs. Sharma guided them through mindfulness exercises, teaching them to embrace the present moment and let go of worries that burdened their minds.

Through meditation and controlled breathing, the residents discovered a profound sense of calm. They realized that they held the power to reduce stress and anxiety, finding solace in the depths of their own being.

Worries about aging, health, and life's uncertainties seemed to melt away as they focused on their breath, embracing the stillness within.

In a world filled with constant distractions, stress, and the demands of modern life, finding balance and inner peace has become a universal quest. As we navigate through the challenges of our fast-paced existence, many of us are turning to yoga—a centuries-old practice that offers a holistic approach to cultivating harmony, physical well-being, and a deeper connection to ourselves.

Yoga, originating in ancient India thousands of years ago, is much more than a physical exercise routine. It is a comprehensive system that encompasses the integration of body, mind, and spirit, leading to profound personal growth and self-realization.

The word "yoga" itself stems from the Sanskrit term "yuj," meaning "to unite" or "to join." It signifies the union of our individual consciousness with the universal consciousness, allowing us to tap into our innate potential and experience a profound sense of wholeness.

At its core, yoga provides a diverse set of tools and techniques designed to foster a balanced and harmonious life.

The practice involves physical postures (asanas) that strengthen, stretch, and purify the body, promoting flexibility, endurance, and vitality.

Through conscious breathing techniques (pranayama), yoga enables practitioners to harness the power of the breath, bringing awareness and control to the life force energy (prana) that flows within us.

By harmonizing the breath, we cultivate a calm and focused mind, relieving stress and promoting mental clarity.

But yoga goes beyond the physical and the breath. It encompasses mindfulness and meditation practices that allow us to quiet the fluctuations of the mind, observe our thoughts and emotions without judgment, and cultivate a deep sense of inner awareness and presence.

Through meditation, we access a state of profound stillness and tap into our inner wisdom, gaining insight and clarity about our true selves and the nature of reality.

The philosophy of yoga extends beyond the mat and into our everyday lives. It offers guiding principles, known as the Yama's (ethical restraints) and niyama's (ethical observances), which provide a moral compass for living a conscious and meaningful life.

These principles, such as non-violence, truthfulness, contentment, self-discipline, and self-study, support our personal growth and guide our interactions with others, promoting harmony within ourselves and in our relationships.

Yoga is a practice that is accessible to everyone, regardless of age, physical ability, or background. It is a journey of self-discovery and self-acceptance, where we learn to listen to our bodies, honor our limitations, and cultivate self-compassion. Yoga encourages us to meet ourselves exactly where we are, embracing our uniqueness and celebrating the diversity of our experiences.

In recent years, yoga has gained widespread popularity worldwide as more and more people recognize its transformative power.

From dedicated yoga studios to community centers and even online platforms, opportunities to explore and deepen your yoga practice abound. Whether you choose to practice alone or in a group setting, the essence of yoga remains the same—a journey of self-exploration, self-care, and self-transformation.

The benefits of yoga are far-reaching and extend beyond the physical.

Regular practice can help reduce stress, improve sleep quality, enhance immune function, increase focus and concentration, and promote emotional well-being. It is a holistic approach to wellness that addresses the interconnectedness of the body, mind, and spirit, nurturing a sense of wholeness and harmony.

As you embark on your own yoga journey, remember that it is a personal and individual practice. There is no competition or comparison in yoga—only self-discovery and growth. Embrace the process with an open heart and an open mind, allowing yourself the space and time to explore the profound depths of your being.

So, whether you seek physical fitness, mental clarity, emotional balance, or spiritual awakening, yoga offers a transformative path to well-being and self-realization. It is an invitation to reconnect with yourself, find stillness amidst the chaos, and discover the profound wisdom that resides within.

Welcome to the world of yoga—a journey of self-discovery, transformation, and the realization of your highest potential.

CHAPTER ONE

Yoga for Seniors Over 50 Benefits

Enhancing Physical Flexibility and Strength:

One of the primary benefits of practicing yoga for older adults is its ability to improve flexibility and increase strength. As we age, our muscles tend to become stiff and less pliable, making simple tasks challenging. Regular participation in yoga sessions helps older individuals improve their range of motion, alleviate joint stiffness, and enhance overall flexibility. Gentle stretches and yoga poses promote muscle tone and strengthen the body, leading to improved balance and reduced risk of falls.

Promoting Joint Health:

Arthritis and other age-related joint issues are common among older adults, often causing discomfort and limiting mobility. Fortunately, yoga offers a low-impact exercise option that can alleviate joint pain and stiffness. Through gentle movements and specific poses, yoga can lubricate the joints, improve their mobility, and reduce inflammation.

Moreover, practicing yoga regularly can help mitigate the progression of degenerative joint diseases, thereby enhancing the overall joint health of older individuals.

Enhancing Balance and Preventing Falls:

Loss of balance and falls pose significant risks for older adults. These incidents can result in severe injuries, diminished confidence, and reduced independence. Yoga can play a pivotal role in improving balance and stability. By incorporating standing poses, balance exercises, and core strengthening postures, yoga helps older individuals develop a stronger sense of balance and coordination. Increased stability translates into reduced fall risk and improved overall physical confidence.

Boosting Cognitive Function:

Among older adults, cognitive deterioration brought on by age is a widespread worry. However, research suggests that engaging in regular physical and mental exercises can help preserve cognitive function. Yoga combines physical movement with mindfulness and breath control, stimulating brain activity and enhancing mental clarity. Regular yoga practice has been shown to improve memory, focus, and attention span. Additionally, the mind-body connection fostered by yoga can have a positive impact on mental well-being, reducing stress, anxiety, and depression.

Managing Chronic Conditions:

Yoga offers immense benefits for managing chronic health conditions that often accompany aging, such as hypertension, diabetes, and cardiovascular diseases. Numerous studies have shown that yoga can help regulate blood pressure, improve blood circulation, and enhance cardiovascular health. Additionally, practicing yoga promotes weight management and can assist in blood sugar regulation. By incorporating yoga into their routine, older adults can gain better control over chronic conditions, leading to an improved overall quality of life.

Fostering Emotional Well-being and Stress Reduction:

In addition to its physical benefits, yoga has a profound impact on emotional well-being and stress reduction. Older adults often face unique challenges, such as the loss of loved ones, retirement, or a decline in physical abilities. These changes can lead to feelings of loneliness, anxiety, and depression. Yoga offers a therapeutic outlet for addressing these emotional concerns.

The practice of yoga encourages mindfulness and self-awareness, allowing individuals to connect with their inner selves and cultivate a sense of peace and calm. Through deep breathing exercises, meditation, and relaxation techniques, yoga helps reduce stress, alleviate anxiety, and promote a positive outlook on life. Moreover, the social aspect of attending yoga classes provides older adults with a supportive community, fostering a sense of belonging and combating feelings of isolation.

Improving Sleep Quality:

Sleep disturbances are common among older adults, often resulting from factors such as hormonal changes, medical conditions, or anxiety. Poor sleep can have a detrimental impact on overall health and well-being. Yoga can play a valuable role in improving sleep quality for older individuals. By practicing gentle yoga poses, breathing exercises, and relaxation techniques before bedtime, the body and mind can enter a state of deep relaxation, promoting better sleep patterns. Yoga helps release tension and calms the nervous system, allowing for a more restful and rejuvenating sleep.

Cultivating Mindfulness and Self-Acceptance:

Yoga encourages individuals to be present in the moment and develop a mindful awareness of their bodies, thoughts, and emotions. For older adults, this can be particularly powerful in fostering self-acceptance and embracing the aging process. By practicing yoga, older individuals can learn to appreciate and honor their bodies, focusing on what they can do rather than what they may have lost. This mindset shift promotes self-esteem, resilience, and a positive attitude towards the aging process.

Social Engagement and Community Connection:

Engaging in yoga classes or group sessions provides older adults with an opportunity to connect with like-minded individuals, fostering social interaction and community engagement. Participating in yoga classes encourages friendship, support, and a sense of belonging. The supportive environment created within yoga communities can be especially beneficial for older adults who may be experiencing feelings of loneliness or isolation.

The social aspect of yoga can contribute to overall mental well-being and provide a valuable support system.

A Lifelong Practice:

One of the most significant advantages of yoga for older adults is its adaptability and suitability for all fitness levels. Whether an individual is a beginner or has been practicing yoga for years, the practice can be tailored to meet their specific needs and abilities. Yoga offers a low-impact and gentle form of exercise that can be modified to accommodate physical limitations or health conditions. This inclusivity makes yoga a lifelong practice that older adults can continue to enjoy and benefit from well into their golden years.

Yoga holds immense potential for improving the physical, mental, and emotional well-being of older adults. Its gentle yet effective approach offers numerous benefits, including enhanced flexibility, joint health, balance, cognitive function, chronic disease management, emotional well-being, and sleep quality.

Additionally, yoga provides a supportive community, fosters mindfulness, and promotes self-acceptance.

As older adults embrace yoga as part of their regular routine, they can experience a greater sense of vitality, improved overall quality of life, and a deeper connection between mind, body, and spirit. So, roll out the mat and embark on a journey to health, happiness, and harmony through the practice of yoga.

7 Day Yoga for Seniors Over 50 Meal Plan

Day 1

Breakfast:

Quinoa Porridge

Ingredients:

- 1/2 cup quinoa
- 1 cup of non-dairy milk, such as almond milk
- 1 tablespoon honey or maple syrup
- Fresh berries for topping

Preparation:

1. Rinse quinoa thoroughly and cook according to package instructions with almond milk.

2. Once cooked, stir in honey or maple syrup.

3. Top with fresh berries.

Lunch:

Chickpea Salad Wrap

Ingredients:

- 1 cup canned chickpeas, rinsed and drained

- 1/4 cup diced cucumber

- 1/4 cup diced bell pepper

- 1/4 cup diced tomato

- 2 tablespoons chopped fresh parsley

- 1 tablespoon lemon juice

- Salt and pepper to taste

- Whole grain tortilla wrap

Preparation:

1. In a bowl, combine chickpeas, cucumber, bell pepper, tomato, parsley, lemon juice, salt, and pepper.

2. Mash some of the chickpeas to create a chunky texture.

3. Spread the mixture onto a whole grain tortilla, wrap tightly, and cut in half.

Dinner:

Baked Salmon with Steamed Vegetables

Ingredients:

- 4 oz salmon fillet

- 1 tablespoon olive oil

- 1/2 teaspoon lemon zest

- 1 teaspoon lemon juice

- Salt and pepper to taste

- Assorted steamed vegetables (e.g., broccoli, carrots, cauliflower)

Preparation:

1. Preheat the oven to 375°F (190°C).

2. Rub the salmon fillet with olive oil, lemon zest, lemon juice, salt, and pepper.

3. Place the salmon on a baking sheet and bake for 12-15 minutes, or until cooked through.

4. Serve with a side of steamed vegetables.

Day 2

Breakfast:

Overnight Chia Pudding

Ingredients:

1. 2 tablespoons chia seeds

2. 1 cup of non-dairy milk, such as almond milk

3. 1 tablespoon honey or maple syrup

4. Sliced almonds and fresh fruits for topping

Preparation:

1. In a bowl or jar, mix chia seeds, almond milk, and honey/maple syrup.

2. Stir well and refrigerate overnight.

3. In the morning, give it a good stir and top with sliced almonds and fresh fruits.

Lunch:

Quinoa Salad with Roasted Vegetables

Ingredients:

- 1 cup cooked quinoa

- 1 cup roasted vegetables (e.g., zucchini, eggplant, bell peppers)

- 2 tablespoons chopped fresh basil

- 1 tablespoon lemon juice

- 1 tablespoon olive oil

- Salt and pepper to taste

Preparation:

1. Combine cooked quinoa, roasted vegetables, basil, lemon juice, extra virgin olive oil, salt, and pepper in a big bowl.

2. Mix well and, if necessary, adjust the seasoning.

Dinner:

Vegetable Stir-Fry with Tofu

Ingredients:

- 1 cup tofu, cubed

- 1 tablespoon sesame oil

- 2 cups mixed stir-fry vegetables (e.g., broccoli, snap peas, bell peppers, mushrooms)

- 2 tablespoons low-sodium soy sauce

- 1 tablespoon rice vinegar

- 1 teaspoon honey or maple syrup

- Cooked brown rice or quinoa (optional, as a side)

Preparation:

1. In a big skillet, warm the sesame oil over medium heat.

2. Add tofu and cook until lightly browned.

3. Add stir-fry vegetables and cook until tender-crisp.

4. Mix the soy sauce, rice vinegar, and honey/maple syrup in a small bowl. Pour over the vegetables and tofu, stirring well to coat.

5. If desired, serve the dish with cooked brown rice or quinoa.

Day 3

Breakfast:

Oatmeal with Berries and Almonds

Ingredients:

- 1/2 cup rolled oats
- 1 cup water
- 1/2 cup almond milk (or any non-dairy milk)
- Fresh berries
- Sliced almonds
- 1 tablespoon honey or maple syrup (optional)

Preparation:

1. In a saucepan, combine rolled oats, water, and almond milk.

2. Boil for a moment, then turn down the heat and simmer for five minutes, stirring now and then.

3. After taking it off the heat, wait a minute.

4. Top with fresh berries, sliced almonds, and a drizzle of honey or maple syrup if desired.

Lunch:

Lentil Soup

Ingredients:

- 1 cup red lentils, rinsed and drained

- 1 onion, chopped

- 2 carrots, diced

- 2 celery stalks, diced

- 2 garlic cloves, minced

- 4 cups vegetable broth

- 1 teaspoon ground cumin

- 1 teaspoon ground coriander

- 1/2 teaspoon turmeric

- Salt and pepper to taste

Preparation:

1. In a large pot, sauté onion, carrots, celery, and garlic until softened.

2. Add lentils, vegetable broth, cumin, coriander, turmeric, salt, and pepper.

3. When the lentils are ready, simmer for about 20 minutes after bringing to a boil.

4. Adjust the seasoning if needed.

Dinner:

Grilled Chicken Breast with Roasted Sweet Potatoes

Ingredients:

- 4 oz chicken breast

- 1 tablespoon olive oil

- 1/2 teaspoon dried rosemary

- 1/2 teaspoon dried thyme

- Salt and pepper to taste

- 1 large sweet potato, cubed

- 1 tablespoon melted coconut oil

- 1/2 teaspoon paprika

- Steamed green beans (as a side)

Preparation:

1. Preheat the grill or grill pan.

2. Rub chicken breast with olive oil, dried rosemary, dried thyme, salt, and pepper.

3. Grill the chicken for about 6-8 minutes per side, or until cooked through.

4. Meanwhile, preheat the oven to 400°F (200°C).

5. In a bowl, toss sweet potato cubes with melted coconut oil, paprika, salt, and pepper.

6. Spread sweet potatoes on a baking sheet and roast for 25-30 minutes, or until tender.

7. Serve the grilled chicken with roasted sweet potatoes and steamed green beans.

Day 4

Breakfast:

Yogurt Parfait

Ingredients:

- 1 cup plain Greek yogurt

- 1/4 cup granola

- 1/4 cup mixed berries

- 1 tablespoon honey or maple syrup (optional)

Preparation:

1. In a glass or bowl, layer Greek yogurt, granola, mixed berries, and drizzle with honey or maple syrup if desired.

Lunch:

Spinach and Feta Salad

Ingredients:

- 2 cups fresh spinach leaves

- 1/4 cup crumbled feta cheese

- 1/4 cup sliced red onions

- 1/4 cup cherry tomatoes, halved

- 2 tablespoons toasted pine nuts

- 1 tablespoon balsamic vinegar

- 1 tablespoon extra-virgin olive oil

- Salt and pepper to taste

Preparation:

1. In a large bowl, combine spinach, feta cheese, red onions, cherry tomatoes, and toasted pine nuts.

2. Drizzle with balsamic vinegar and olive oil.

3. Mix thoroughly after adding salt and pepper to taste.

Dinner:

Lentil and Vegetable Curry

Ingredients:

- 1 cup cooked lentils

- 1 tablespoon coconut oil

- 1 onion, chopped

- 2 cloves garlic, minced

- 1 tablespoon grated fresh ginger

- 1 tablespoon curry powder

- 1 teaspoon ground cumin

- 1 teaspoon ground turmeric

- 1 cup diced tomatoes

- 1 cup vegetable broth

- 2 cups mixed vegetables (e.g., cauliflower, peas, carrots)

- 1/4 cup chopped fresh cilantro

- Cooked brown rice (optional, as a side)

Preparation:

1. In a sizable skillet or pot, warm the coconut oil over medium heat.

2. Add onion, garlic, and ginger. Sauté until fragrant and softened.

3. Stir in curry powder, cumin, and turmeric. Cook for 1 minute.

4. Add diced tomatoes and vegetable broth. Bring to a simmer.

5. Add mixed vegetables and cooked lentils. Vegetables should be cooked till soft under cover.

6. Stir in fresh cilantro.

7. Serve with cooked brown rice if desired.

Day 5

Breakfast:

Vegetable Omelet

Ingredients:

- 2 eggs

- 1/4 cup chopped bell peppers

- 1/4 cup diced tomatoes

- 1/4 cup diced mushrooms

- 2 tablespoons chopped fresh parsley

- Salt and pepper to taste

- 1 teaspoon olive oil

Preparation:

1. In a bowl, whisk eggs with bell peppers, tomatoes, mushrooms, parsley, salt, and pepper.

2. In a non-stick skillet, warm up the olive oil over medium heat.

3. Cook the egg mixture until set in the skillet after pouring it in.

4. Cook for another minute after flipping the omelet.

5. Serve hot.

Lunch:

Caprese Salad

Ingredients:

- 1 large ripe tomato, sliced

- 4 oz fresh mozzarella cheese, sliced

- Fresh basil leaves

- 1 tablespoon balsamic vinegar

- 1 tablespoon extra-virgin olive oil

- Salt and pepper to taste

Preparation:

1. Arrange tomato slices and fresh mozzarella slices on a plate.

2. Tuck fresh basil leaves in between.

3. Drizzle with balsamic vinegar and olive oil.

4. Season with salt and pepper.

Dinner:

Grilled Shrimp Skewers with Quinoa Salad

Ingredients:

- 4 oz shrimp, peeled and deveined

- 1 tablespoon olive oil

- 1 clove garlic, minced

- 1 teaspoon lemon zest

- Salt and pepper to taste

- 1/2 cup cooked quinoa

- 1/4 cup diced cucumbers

- 1/4 cup diced red bell peppers

- 2 tablespoons chopped fresh parsley

- 1 tablespoon lemon juice

- 1 tablespoon extra-virgin olive oil

Preparation:

1. Preheat the grill or grill pan.

2. In a bowl, combine shrimp, olive oil, minced garlic, lemon zest, salt, and pepper.

3. Thread the shrimp onto skewers and grill for 2-3 minutes per side, or until cooked through.

4. In another bowl, mix cooked quinoa, cucumbers, red bell peppers, parsley, lemon juice, and extra-virgin olive oil.

5. Serve the grilled shrimp skewers with quinoa salad.

Day 6

Breakfast:

Banana Protein Smoothie

Ingredients:

- 1 ripe banana

- 1 cup of non-dairy milk, such as almond milk

- 1 scoop protein powder (vanilla or your preferred flavor)

- 1 tablespoon almond butter

- 1/2 teaspoon honey or maple syrup (optional)

Preparation:

1. In a blender, combine ripe banana, almond milk, protein powder, almond butter, and honey/maple syrup.

2. Blend until smooth and creamy.

3. Serve chilled.

Lunch:

Quinoa Stuffed Bell Peppers

Ingredients:

- 2 large bell peppers (any color), halved and seeds removed

- 1 cup cooked quinoa

- 1/2 cup black beans, rinsed and drained

- 1/4 cup corn kernels

- 1/4 cup diced tomatoes

- 1/4 cup diced red onions

- 2 tablespoons chopped fresh cilantro

- 1 tablespoon lime juice

- 1/2 teaspoon ground cumin

- Salt and pepper to taste

Preparation:

1. Preheat the oven to 375°F (190°C).

2. In a bowl, mix cooked quinoa, black beans, corn kernels, tomatoes, red onions, cilantro, lime juice, cumin, salt, and pepper.

3. Fill the bell pepper halves with the quinoa mixture.

4. Place the stuffed bell peppers on a baking sheet and bake for 20-25 minutes, or until the peppers are tender.

Dinner:

Baked Cod with Lemon Herb Sauce and Roasted Vegetables

Ingredients:

- 4 oz cod fillet

- 1 tablespoon olive oil

- 1/2 teaspoon dried dill

- 1/2 teaspoon dried thyme

- Salt and pepper to taste

- 1 lemon, sliced

- Assorted roasted vegetables (e.g., Brussels sprouts, asparagus, carrots)

Preparation:

1. Preheat the oven to 375°F (190°C).

2. Rub the cod fillet with olive oil, dried dill, dried thyme, salt, and pepper.

3. Place the cod on a baking sheet and top with lemon slices.

4. Bake the fish for 15 to 20 minutes, or until it is well done.

5. Serve with a side of roasted vegetables.

Day 7

Breakfast:

Veggie Scramble

Ingredients:

- 2 eggs

- 1/4 cup diced bell peppers

- 1/4 cup diced zucchini

- 1/4 cup diced mushrooms

- 1/4 cup diced tomatoes

- 2 tablespoons chopped fresh spinach

- Salt and pepper to taste

- 1 teaspoon olive oil

Preparation:

1. In a bowl, whisk eggs with bell peppers, zucchini, mushrooms, tomatoes, spinach, salt, and pepper.

2. In a non-stick skillet, warm up the olive oil over medium heat.

3. Scramble the egg mixture in the skillet until it is fully cooked.

4. Serve hot.

Lunch:

Chickpea and Vegetable Curry

Ingredients:

- 1 cup canned chickpeas, rinsed and drained

- 1 tablespoon coconut oil

- 1 onion, chopped

- 2 cloves garlic, minced

- 1 tablespoon grated fresh ginger

- 1 tablespoon curry powder

- 1 teaspoon ground cumin

- 1/2 teaspoon ground turmeric

- 1 cup diced tomatoes

- 1 cup coconut milk

- 2 cups mixed vegetables (e.g., cauliflower, peas, carrots)

- 1/4 cup chopped fresh cilantro

- Cooked brown rice or quinoa (optional, as a side)

Preparation:

1. In a sizable skillet or pot, warm the coconut oil over medium heat.

2. Add onion, garlic, and ginger. Sauté until fragrant and softened.

3. Stir in curry powder, cumin, and turmeric. Cook for 1 minute.

4. Add diced tomatoes, coconut milk, and mixed vegetables. Simmer until the vegetables are tender.

5. Stir in chickpeas and fresh cilantro.

6. If desired, serve the dish with cooked brown rice or quinoa.

Dinner:

Baked Chicken Thighs with Roasted Potatoes and Steamed Broccoli

Ingredients:

- 2 chicken thighs, bone-in and skin-on

- 1 tablespoon olive oil

- 1 teaspoon dried thyme

- 1 teaspoon paprika

- Salt and pepper to taste

- 2 medium-sized potatoes, cubed

- 1 tablespoon melted coconut oil

- 1/2 teaspoon garlic powder

- Steamed broccoli (as a side)

Preparation:

1. Preheat the oven to 400°F (200°C).

2. Rub chicken thighs with olive oil, dried thyme, paprika, salt, and pepper.

3. Place the chicken on a baking sheet and bake for 25-30 minutes, or until the chicken is cooked through and the skin is crispy.

4. Meanwhile, in a bowl, toss cubed potatoes with melted coconut oil, garlic powder, salt, and pepper.

5. Spread potatoes on a separate baking sheet and roast for 20-25 minutes, or until golden and crispy.

6. Serve the baked chicken thighs with roasted potatoes and steamed broccoli.

CHAPTER TWO

Yoga Exercises for Seniors and How to do Them

1. Mountain Pose (Tad asana):

Instructions:

1. Stand with feet hip-width apart, arms relaxed by your sides.

2. Engage your abdominal muscles and elongate your spine.

3. Take deep breaths, feeling grounded and stable.

2. Chair Pose (Utkatasana):

Instructions:

1. Stand with feet together, arms extended overhead.

2. As though settling back into a chair, bending your knees.

3. Keep your chest lifted and core engaged.

3. Warrior I (Virabhadrasana I):

Instructions:

1. Step one foot back, keeping both feet facing forward.

2. Bend your front knee, keeping it aligned with your ankle.

3. Raise your arms overhead, keeping your shoulders relaxed.

4. Warrior II (Virabhadrasana II):

Instructions:

1. From Warrior I, open your hips and extend your arms out to the sides.

2. Keep your front knee bent and gaze forward over your front hand.

3. Engage your core and breathe deeply.

5. Tree Pose (Vrikshasana):

Instructions:

1. Stand with feet hip-width apart, shift your weight onto one foot.

2. Put the sole of the opposite foot on your calf or inner thigh.

3. Find your balance, bring your hands together at your heart.

6. Triangle Pose (Trikonasana):

Instructions:

1. Stand with legs wide apart.

7. Child's Pose (Balasana):

Instructions:

1. Kneel on the floor, sit back on your heels, and lower your forehead to the mat.

2. Put your arms out in front of or next to your body.

3. Relax and breathe deeply, feeling a gentle stretch in your lower back.

8. Cat-Cow Pose (Marjaryasana-Bitilasana):

Instructions:

1. Start on all fours with your knees under your hips and your hands under your shoulders.

2. Inhale, arch your back, and lift your tailbone and head (Cow Pose).

3. Exhale, round your spine and tuck your chin (Cat Pose).

4. Alternate between the two poses, syncing movement with your breath.

9. Downward Facing Dog (Adho Mukha Svanasana):

Instructions:

1. Beginning on all fours, lift your hips back and up to create an inverted V shape.

2. Press your palms and heels into the floor, lengthening your spine.

3. Breathe deeply and relax your neck and head.

10. Bridge Pose (Setu Bandhasana):

Instructions:

1. Knees bent and feet hip-width apart, lie on your back.

2. Press your feet into the floor, lift your hips, and interlace your hands beneath your back.

3. Hold the pose for a few breaths, engaging your glutes and thighs.

11. Pose with the Legs Up the Wall (Viparita Karani):

Instructions:

1. Sit sideways close to a wall, then swing your legs up against the wall as you lie back.

2. With your palms facing up, place your arms at your sides.

3. Relax and breathe deeply, enjoying the gentle stretch in your legs.

12. Seated Forward Bend (Paschimottanasana):

Instructions:

1. Stretch your legs out in front of you as you sit on the ground.

2. Reach forward, lengthening your spine, and gently fold forward from the hips.

3. Breathe deeply while holding onto your shins, ankles, or feet.

13. Cobra Pose (Bhujangasana):

Instructions:

1. Lie on your belly, legs extended and tops of your feet pressing into the floor.

2. Place your hands beside your shoulders, elbows close to your body.

3. Inhale, lift your chest off the floor while keeping your pelvis grounded.

14. Seated Spinal Twist (Ardha Matsyendrasana):

Instructions:

1. Sit with legs extended, bend one knee, and place the foot on the floor outside the opposite thigh.

2. Place your opposite elbow on the outer side of the bent knee and gently twist.

3. Keep your spine long and breathe deeply, then switch sides.

15. Warrior III (Virabhadrasana III):

Instructions:

1. Stand with feet hip-width apart, shift your weight onto one foot.

2. Hinge forward at the hips, extend the other leg straight behind you.

3. Reach your arms forward or place your hands on your hips for balance.

16. Happy Baby Pose (Ananda Balasana):

Instructions:

1. Lie on your back and draw your knees toward your chest.

2. Reach for the inside edges of your feet and open your knees.

3. Gently rock side to side, releasing tension in your lower back.

17. Reclining Bound Angle Pose (Supta Baddha Konasana):

Instructions:

1. Bring your feet's soles together as you lay on your back, letting your knees droop.

2. Place your arms alongside your body or rest your hands on your belly.

3. Relax and take slow, deep breaths, allowing your hips to open.

18. Mountain Pose with Arm Variation:

Instructions:

1. Stand with feet hip-width apart, interlace your fingers behind your back.

2. Straighten your arms and lift them away from your body, feeling a stretch in your chest and shoulders.

3. Lengthen your spine and breathe deeply.

19. Standing Forward Bend (Uttanasana):

Instructions:

1. Stand with feet hip-width apart, hinge forward from your hips, and let your head and arms hang.

2. Bend your knees as much as needed to maintain a comfortable stretch.

3. Breathe deeply and relax your shoulders and neck.

20. Sphinx Pose:

Instructions:

1. Lie on your belly, place your forearms on the mat, elbows under your shoulders.

2. Press your forearms and palms into the floor, lift your chest, and relax your shoulders.

3. Keep your neck long and gaze forward, breathing steadily.

21. Half Moon Pose (Ardha Chandrasana):

Instructions:

1. Stand with feet together, lift one leg off the ground, and place the foot on your calf or thigh.

2. Extend your arms overhead, interlace your fingers, and extend your index fingers upward.

3. Find your balance and breathe deeply, then switch sides.

22. Warrior I with Chair Support:

Instructions:

1. Place your feet hip-width apart as you stance behind a chair.

2. Step one foot back, keeping both feet facing forward.

3. Bend your front knee while holding onto the chair for support.

23. Supine Spinal Twist:

Instructions:

1. Lie on your back, bend your knees, and extend your arms out to the sides.

2. While maintaining your shoulders firmly planted, bend your knees to one side.

3. Turn your head in the opposite direction and breathe deeply.

24. Supported Bridge Pose:

Instructions:

1. Knees bent and feet flat on the floor, lie on your back.

2. For support, place a folded blanket or bolster beneath your hips.

3. Lift your hips off the floor, keeping your shoulders and head grounded.

25. Supported Shoulderstand (Salamba Sarvangasana):

Instructions:

1. Place a folded blanket or bolster under your shoulders and upper back.

2. Your legs should be raised up toward the ceiling as you lay on your back.

3. Support your lower back with your hands and keep your gaze towards your toes.

26. Supported Headstand (Salamba Sirsasana):

Instructions:

1. Stand facing a wall with your forearms resting on the floor.

2. Interlace your fingers and place them on the floor, creating a triangle with your forearms.

3. Place the top of your head on the floor and walk your feet towards your head.

27. Butterfly Pose (Baddha Konasana):

Instructions:

1. Put your feet together and sit down on the ground.

2. Hold onto your feet or ankles and gently press your knees toward the floor.

3. Sit tall and breathe deeply, feeling a stretch in your inner thighs.

28. Corpse Pose (Savasana):

Instructions:

1. With your hands facing up, lie on your back with your arms at your sides.

2. Allow your body to unwind completely while closing your eyes.

3. Let go of any tension in your muscles and focus on deep, slow breathing.

4. Stay in this pose for several minutes, enjoying a state of deep relaxation.

29. Standing Side Stretch:

Instructions:

1. Standing with your feet hip-width apart, extend your arms in front of you.

2. Interlace your fingers and invert your palms.

3. Lean gently to one side, lengthening the opposite
   side of your body.

4. Deeply inhale, then repeat on the opposite side.

30. Garland Pose (Malasana):

Instructions:

1. Stand with feet wider than hip-width apart, toes
   turned out slightly.

2. Squat down, keeping your heels on the ground if
   possible.

3. Bring your palms together at your heart, pressing
   your elbows against your inner thighs.

4. Breathe deeply and feel a stretch in your hips and
   groin.

31. Camel Pose (Ustrasana):

Instructions:

1. Kneel on the ground, keeping your legs hip distance
   apart.

2. With your fingers pointed down, place your hands on your lower back.

3. Arch your back and lean backward, lifting your chest and gazing toward the ceiling.

4. Breathe deeply and engage your core.

32. Reclined Twist:

Instructions:

1. Lay on your back with your arms outstretched.

2. Bend one knee and cross it over the opposite leg, allowing it to rest on the floor.

3. Gently lower your crossed legs to one side, turning your head in the opposite direction.

4. Deeply inhale, then repeat on the opposite side.

33. Supported Fish Pose:

Instructions:

1. Sit with legs extended in front of you and place a bolster or rolled-up blanket behind you.

2. Lie back over the bolster, supporting your head and upper back.

3. Relax your arms by your sides and breathe deeply, opening your chest.

34. Eagle Pose (Garudasana):

Instructions:

1. Stand with your arms by your sides and your feet hip-width apart.

2. Bend your knees slightly and cross one leg over the other, wrapping the foot around the calf if possible.

3. Cross your arms in front of your body, bringing your elbows to shoulder height.

4. Breathe deeply and switch sides.

35. Supine Hand-to-Big-Toe Pose:

Instructions:

1. One leg should be raised straight up toward the ceiling as you lay on your back.

2. Hold onto the back of your thigh or calf, or use a strap if needed.

3. Relax your shoulders and breathe deeply, feeling a stretch in your hamstrings.

4. Switch legs and repeat.

36. Gate Pose (Parighasana):

Instructions:

1. Kneel down on the ground and join your legs.

2. Extend one leg out to the side and keep the other knee on the ground.

3. Raise your arms overhead, then bend sideways towards the extended leg.

4. Deeply inhale, then repeat on the opposite side.

37. Supported Pigeon Pose:

Instructions:

1. Start on all fours, bring one knee forward, and place it behind your wrist.

2. Slide the opposite leg back, straightening it behind you.

3. For support, place a bolster or folded blanket beneath your hips.

4. Relax your upper body and breathe deeply, feeling a stretch in your hip.

38. Standing Forward Bend with Support:

Instructions:

1. Stand with feet hip-width apart, holding onto a sturdy chair or countertop.

2. Allow your upper body to hang and hinge forward from your hips.

3. Keep a slight bend in your knees if needed and breathe deeply, releasing tension in your back.

39. Extended Triangle Pose (Utthita Trikonasana):

Instructions:

1. Stand with feet wide apart, turn one foot out 90 degrees and the other foot slightly in.

2. Extend your arms out to the sides, then bend at the hip towards the extended leg.

3. Place your hand on your shin, ankle, or the floor, and reach the other arm toward the ceiling.

4. Deeply inhale, then repeat on the opposite side.

40. Supported Warrior III:

Instructions:

1. Stand behind a chair or hold onto a wall for support.

2. Shift your weight onto one foot and extend the opposite leg straight back.

3. Lean your torso forward while keeping your back leg lifted and parallel to the floor.

4. Find your balance, engage your core, and breathe deeply.

CONCLUSION

In conclusion, yoga for seniors over 50 is an invaluable practice that promotes physical well-being, mental clarity, and emotional balance. It offers a wide range of benefits that can significantly enhance the quality of life for this age group. Throughout this discussion, we have explored the various aspects of yoga that make it particularly suitable for seniors, such as its adaptability, gentle nature, and emphasis on mindfulness and self-care.

One of the key advantages of yoga for seniors is its ability to improve physical strength, flexibility, and balance. As we age, our bodies naturally undergo changes that can lead to decreased mobility and increased risk of falls.

However, engaging in regular yoga practice can counteract these effects by stretching and strengthening muscles, improving joint mobility, and enhancing overall balance and stability. By maintaining a strong and supple body, seniors can continue to perform daily activities with ease and confidence, ultimately promoting independence and a higher quality of life.

Furthermore, yoga provides a powerful tool for mental and emotional well-being. Seniors often face unique challenges such as transitioning into retirement, dealing with loss, and coping with health issues. Yoga offers a supportive environment that encourages self-reflection, stress reduction, and the cultivation of inner peace. Through mindful movement, breathing exercises, and meditation, seniors can develop greater self-awareness, manage stress more effectively, and find solace in the present moment. These practices can lead to improved mood, reduced anxiety and depression, and an overall sense of calm and contentment.

Additionally, yoga fosters a sense of community and connection among seniors. Participating in group classes or joining yoga communities allows individuals to engage in social interactions, build relationships, and share their journey with like-minded peers. This sense of belonging and camaraderie can be particularly beneficial for seniors who may experience feelings of isolation or loneliness. By coming together in a supportive environment, seniors can find a sense of belonging, develop new friendships, and experience the power of human connection.

Moreover, yoga is a holistic practice that addresses the interconnectedness of the mind, body, and spirit. It encourages seniors to embrace self-care and prioritize their well-being on all levels. Through regular yoga practice, seniors can develop a greater sense of self-compassion, acceptance, and gratitude. By nurturing the mind-body connection, they can cultivate a deeper understanding and appreciation of their own bodies and their unique capabilities. This newfound awareness can lead to increased self-esteem, self-confidence, and an overall positive outlook on life.

In conclusion, yoga for seniors over 50 is a transformative practice that offers a multitude of physical, mental, and emotional benefits. It empowers seniors to take an active role in their well-being and provides them with the tools to navigate the aging process with grace and resilience.

By incorporating yoga into their lives, seniors can enjoy improved physical strength and flexibility, enhanced mental clarity and emotional balance, and a greater sense of connection and community.

As a gentle yet powerful practice, yoga has the potential to unlock new levels of vitality, peace, and joy for seniors as they embrace the later stages of life.

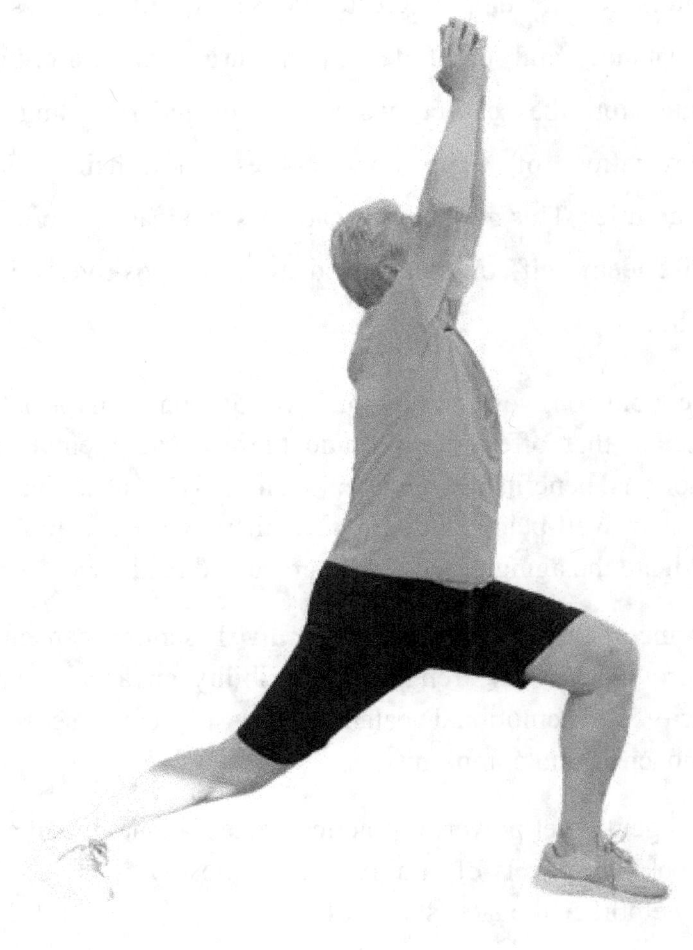

www.ingramcontent.com/pod-product-compliance
Lightning Source LLC
Chambersburg PA
CBHW070958250726

48663CB00002B/284